INTERACTIVE GUIDE
FOR *Women*

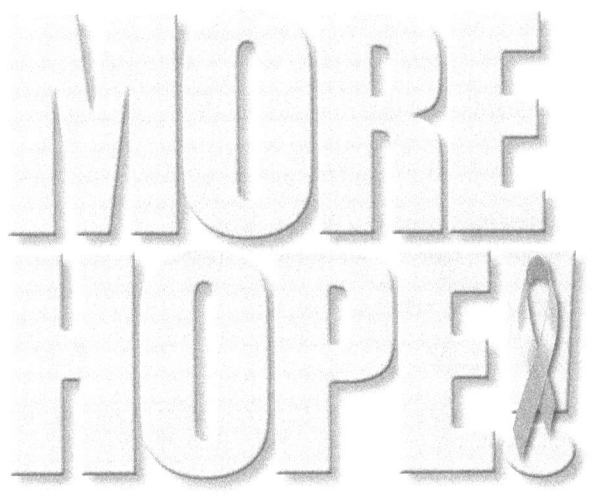

MORE HOPE!
emerging...
FROM THE SHADOW OF BREAST CANCER

Andrea Hunter
Beth Webb
with Jonathan Hunter

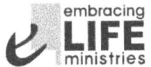

Copyright © 2015 by Andrea Hunter, Beth Webb, Jonathan Hunter

More Hope!
Emerging from the Shadow of Breast Cancer
by Andrea Hunter, Beth Webb, Jonathan Hunter

Printed in the United States of America.

ISBN 9781498450904

All rights reserved solely by the author. The author guarantees all contents are original and do not infringe upon the legal rights of any other person or work. No part of the book may be reproduced or transmitted in any form or by any means electronic or mechanical, including photocopying, recording or by any information storage and retrieval system without written permission of the author. The views expressed in this book are not necessarily those of the publisher.

Scripture quotations taken from the New International Version (NIV). Copyright © 1973, 1978, 1984, 2011 by Biblica, Inc.™. Used by permission. All rights reserved.

When quoting authors' work or the Bible we have respected their/its particular capitalization in reference to deity.

Cover design: mdr design   www.mdr1.com

Book design Xulon Press

www.xulonpress.com

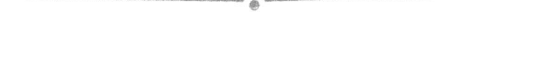

The thief comes only to steal and kill and destroy; I have come that they may have life, and have it to the full.

John 10:10

Acknowledgments

Our heartfelt appreciation to the courageous women who have faced down death, emerged from the shadows of cancer, and continue to shine the light of hope. Special recognition to Anthonie Meister, Cindy Martin, Elizabeth Schmus, Hadassah Lozano, Terry Taylor, and Patti Yung, as well as artist and author Jean Shen (who wrote Out of the Wilderness, My Healing Journey through Cancer and Cancerous Lies). **More Hope!** *is richer for their contributions, wisdom, and experience. Additional thanks to Jim Wilder and the folks at Life Model Works: Our "Time to Connect to Hope" is in part inspired by their small group publications.*

Contents

Acknowledgments vii
Table of Contents ix
About the Authors xi
Introduction: By Jonathan Hunter xv

Session One: Hope–Your Story 1
Session Two: Hope–Reclaiming Your Identity and
    Dreams (before and after cancer) 9
Session Three: Hope–Faith, and Peace in
    Treatment Choices. 17
Session Four: Hope–Inviting Jesus into Your Weakness 27
Session Five: Hope–Emerging from the Shadow of
    Breast Cancer (The Prayer). 35
Session Six: Hope–Embracing God's Community
    of Healing (Testimonies) 43

Appendix I: Journey of Hope! Beth Webb's Story 53
Appendix II: Scriptures of Hope, Healing & Community. . . . 69
Appendix III: God's Truth Destroys Cancerous
    Lies (Table) 77
Appendix IV: Resources for Group Leaders/Facilitators . . . 81

About the Authors and the Booklet

Andrea Hunter
Beth Webb
Jonathan Hunter

This booklet has emerged from the combined healing-group participation, leadership and life experiences of the authors, as well as from the life stories of many courageous women journeying through and out from breast cancer's shadowlands.

Jonathan Hunter founded ARM (the AIDS Resource Ministry) in 1985; as the vision expanded, it would ultimately become Embracing Life Ministries (ELM). Beth Webb, who became the catalyst for this book worked with him as an assistant and associate at that time under the umbrella of Desert Stream Ministries. Andrea Hunter soon joined as a volunteer in what was one of the first Christian ministries to men, women, and children affected by HIV/AIDS. All three were involved in co-hosting support groups and doing home and hospital visitation, as well as training others to do the same. Jonathan and Beth took the experience from the group settings and turned them into the first and most comprehensive ELM resource and foundational exposition of the ministry, the *Embracing Life Series Guidebook*.

Andrea's background in counseling, creative editorial, theology and the arts contributed to her work with ELM and the album *Healing Presence*, which she produced on behalf of the ministry to raise support for outreach. She has also had an active and substantive editorial role in EL's small group "More!" series, beginning with the *More Life!: Breaking Free from the spirit of death* booklet.With a change of name and extended reach, Embracing Life grew to encompass any and all conditions that influence and impact human lives.

Beth transitioned to a new job at Fuller Theological seminary in academic advising in 2002 where she applied the wisdom gained in her studies and life, including her BA from UCLA, and MAT studies at Fuller Theological Seminary to her new position. Suddenly, her life was interrupted by breast cancer. Fuller provided the perfect context for her to reflect on her journey through the disease, accompanied by God and her faith family.

With the Embracing Life team, Jonathan continues to train teams and leaders of churches and para-church organizations around the world to implement the healing net of ELM in their individual context. Books he has written and co-written for the ministry have been translated into many languages. He attends and serves at HRock Church in Pasadena, California.

Beth attends and has served on the vestry at St. Luke's Anglican Church in La Crescenta and is a board member of Embracing Life Ministries. She worked for 15 years at Fuller Theological Seminary, completing her tenure there as director of academic advising. She is cancer-free, and yearly runs 5Ks to raise awareness and support for breast cancer. In her free time, she scales mountain trails, enjoys a good meal and fellowship with friends, and runs the beach at San Clemente whenever she gets the chance.

Andrea Hunter is a member of the Vineyard Christian Community in Aliso Viejo, where she participates as a

About the Authors and the Booklet

support team member in relational healing classes. She is also an ELM board member. After 13 years at Warner Bros. Records, she served at Fuller as the executive assistant to the dean of the School of Psychology for two years and recently completed six years as director of creative/publishing services and senior editor/writer at *Worship Leader* magazine. She has produced (and co-written) four worship CDs.

USING THIS BOOK
The booklet can be read/prayed/journaled on one's own, but is intended for a group context, where its power and truth based on Scripture can be amplified by the experience and wisdom of a community. Be creative when you come together. What is here is only a suggested framework for healing. Utilize discussion sections with freedom.

More Hope! may be presented in various formats. Please go to Appendix IV: Resources for Group Leaders/Facilitators to explore the possibilities for gathering.

Prayers are also included for participants to pray out loud with each other, usually lead by the group facilitator/leader with group members responding. In certain sections, prayerful interaction in pairs is also suggested. ***Note**: Instructions are italicized and prayers are in bold.

For information seminars, trainings, and other healing opportunities or to purchase additional copies of **More Hope!** or any other ELM publication, visit www.embracinglife.us or Xulon press: www.xulonpress.com

Introduction

It seems like everyone has a friend or family member who has faced breast cancer in one form or another. This pervasiveness, unfortunately, has not produced a corresponding response of helpful materials and support groups for *Christian* women to turn to for encouragement, fellowship and healing. Thus, **More Hope!**

This booklet has its roots in an enduring, rich friendship of many years between Beth Webb and me. Our relationship began years ago as co-workers in AIDS ministry and over the years has become more like that of brother and sister. She always renders invaluable counsel and is a faithful, cherished friend indeed!

When Beth first showed me a seminary paper about her breast cancer experience, I was moved and impressed. What made reading it compelling was her disarming, transparent writing style: unabashedly honest about the emotional and spiritual struggles within and frank about what was helpful (or not) when it came to the advice from without.

After reading it, I enthused to Beth that it could make a great guide for small-group work for other Christian women going though the same experience. In spite of my pushy flattery and goads to pursue the booklet thing, it was clearly premature. She wasn't interested, even with my insistence that Embracing Life Ministries publish it. You do with it what you want, but I don't really want to revisit and rework that project, was basically her response. Rightly so, it was *her* experience and *her* testimony after all. Determined as I was, I needed to back off and give the idea time to marinate in her imagination. When I eventually (years later!) came back with a proposal that my sister-in-law Andrea and I take over the project, her reply was "Go for it! It'll be great." Yet, as these things sometimes happen after an appropriate amount of time to reflect, Beth decided to join us in the process. So we're all in it together, now.

While Beth's seminary paper was our primary source in deciding what issues to cover, we also sought out testimonies, through a questionnaire, from other women of varied backgrounds who have also been impacted by breast cancer: marrieds, singles, different ethnicities – all friends and acquaintances. To them we owe much for their heartfelt candor in sharing their experiences with us. We are so very grateful for their integral input found throughout this guide. We have attempted to put together a sensitive and respectful booklet that provides Christian women with thoughtful, compassionate teachings, testimonies and prayers that address some of the deeply, personal issues surrounding breast cancer and its treatment.

Proverbs 13:12 says, "Hope deferred makes the heart sick, but a longing fulfilled is a tree of life." I pray that the hope and healing found in and through the Cross of Christ (*the* "tree of life") woven into this booklet will help fulfill the longing you may have for honest fellowship with like-minded sisters. May it encourage you with hope for the future.

"For I know the plans I have for you," declares the Lord, "plans to prosper you and not to harm you, plans to give you hope and a future." Jeremiah 29:11

– Jonathan

Session One

Hope – Your Story

> *I wait for the LORD, my whole being waits,*
> *and in his word I put my hope.* Psalm 130:5

"I felt a lump." I mentioned matter-of-factly to my friend Erin, driving her home from the airport following Thanksgiving holiday. I was as surprised as she was to hear myself say it. I quickly waved off her solemn concern and changed the subject. She didn't leave the car without being assured I would be "examined by a doctor"… and she didn't mean maybe.

The next day I sat shell-shocked as my physician made a phone call to the breast clinic to get me in for an immediate ultrasound and biopsy. She was "highly concerned"—the lump was "huge." I watched and listened for some reprieve in her insistence. None—there was no room for delay. As I left and drove home, I felt like I was walking underwater, and everyone's voice felt garbled and far away. – Beth Webb

Each of us has a story about our encounter with breast cancer—where and when it began—whatever place we find ourselves in the process of emerging from its shadow. For some it is not a physical reality, but more of a long-term fear based on brushes with breast cancer through friends or family members, or simply as an observer of news-based stories. For others, it is an uncertainty waiting for the return of a biopsy or mammogram. And for some of us the diagnoses is in, but treatment still looms. And lastly, there are those who have concluded the battle, and either feel a certain *finishedness* or a vulnerable apprehension...

This booklet was birthed out of the journey of Beth Webb. In her story she touches on subjects that are important to consider as we battle, not just for our lives, but our entire worldview, our trust in God... and the very meaning of life. We've included an abbreviated version of Beth's paper in Appendix I, and we've included excerpts in select chapters as a catalyst for reflection, discussion and prayer. Also included are contributions from a number of other women who have emerged from the shadow of breast cancer to find renewed hope.

> *My faith in God went into crisis— for the first time as a believer.*

We each react differently to pronouncements regarding breast cancer, whether it concerns us personally, or a loved one. We started the chapter with Beth's response to her diagnosis. Below are more reactions. As we read them, take time to reflect on what your response was and is at this moment.

> *When I heard my cancer diagnosis, I remember feeling a wonderfully profound sense of the Lord's peace that drove out all negativity and fear. My friends told me that cancer was not from the Lord, and that He was going to use my cancer treatment experience for His glory.* – Anthonie Meister

I felt betrayed, and really struggled with trusting the Lord. I was so angry at the Lord. I could not understand why I was not protected from cancer when I had given my life to follow after Him. My faith in God went into crisis—for the first time as a believer, I doubted and wondered about His existence. – Patti Yung

After hearing the diagnosis from the biopsy, I remembered my mind being in a stage of disbelief. It took some days to hit my emotions. One of the main questions that kept coming to my mind was "Why and how had this happened to me?" I knew Who had the answer to my questions. I just knew down deep in my soul and spirit that I needed to draw close to Him. I also knew from my theology that God was not responsible for this cancer. I understood this very well in my mind, and soul. In fact every time I referred to it, I called it "This stupid cancer." – Hadassah Lozano

I was honestly beyond shocked. Many prayed for us. Something that brought me hope was that I felt I had been forewarned by the Lord that I would go through another "feeling like drowning" experience but that he would bring me through it as he had before with the death of my son. – Elizabeth Schmus

I was shopping at Home Goods the afternoon my doctor called to give me my results. May I just say right now that when you are alone and shopping in a store, that's not really the opportune time or place to receive this type of news, especially when the results are that you have cancer again! Where were God's people to comfort me in this moment of despair? I felt a little light-headed as the doctor was talking and looked around for a chair to sit in. The only chair I could find was one that was placed in a small vignette on a display riser. I climbed up and sat in the chair. People stared. I didn't care. I listened to the doctor with tears silently rolling down my face.

I sat there for a few minutes. I felt totally alone and on display. Questions for God raced through my mind. Wasn't once enough? Why do I have to go through this again? It's not fair! Where are you? Don't you know or care what's happening to me? I was angry. I was angry at God and I was angry at my body for betraying me yet again. – Terry Taylor

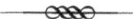

I was told that the lump on my chest was cancer, a part of which was aggressive. My emotions went haywire. I was angry, scared, confused. I wrote in my journal, "My whole life has been in a cocoon of pain and fear from molestation in early childhood, intimidation in schools, a broken marriage (since healed), and then, breast cancer. Cancer is the backdrop for God to teach me to fight as a fierce warrior."
– Jean Shen

We all have a story to tell. Sharing our stories can birth encouragement and hope in each other in ways we might never discover on our own. We want to be named and shaped, not by cancer, but by the God who created us. Each of our stories has to do with who we were uniquely created to be, our history with people and with God, and where we found ourselves confronted by breast cancer. Each of our stories is unique, but in the light of community—shared experience, truth, and deep feeling—hope emerges and we can see beyond the shadows.

Session 1: Hope—Your Story

Questions for Discussion & Reflection

NOTE: *"Time to Connect to Hope" will be repeated each week. The first few minutes of discussion and reflection portion will center on each person asking God to bring to their spirit's attention, "one" thing that happened in the last day, week, month, year, that inspires appreciation, joy, gratitude, or hope. It can be as simple as a moment watching a cloud, or holding a baby, smelling a flower, or sipping coffee. It can be a touch from a loved one or an encounter with God. The leader then offers the opportunity to connect the moment to that week's particular theme.*

- Time to Connect to Hope: *Leader prays out loud, giving group members a moment to reflect:* **God, according to Your wisdom, remind each of us of a "hope" moment during our diagnoses phase or any other moment of hope in our lives where You demonstrated Your love** *(Leader pauses, and instructs the participants to open their eyes when they have seen, heard, or felt something to share). Leader continues:* **Let's take two to three minutes each to share what we saw, felt, or heard and why it inspires hope. If nothing surfaces, then share that. Take a moment to note what God surfaced for you in the Journal section.**

- Where are you in the process of diagnosis? By example:

    o Not diagnosed, but concerned or fearful
    o Just diagnosed.
    o Deciding a course of treatment

- o In treatment
- o Post treatment within first year
- o Post treatment, one or more years

- What are your concerns?

- For those who are post-treatment, how does it feel to revisit the diagnosis phase of your encounter with breast cancer?

- Finally, what are your hopes for this group? *(Take a few minutes each to share your hopes.)*

Prayer
Leader prays out loud in easy to repeat phrases asking participants to follow.

Dear Father: As we come to You, we bring our hopes and fears, our needs and desires. We lay them at Your feet. We trust You to be the light for our path, to show us the way, to bring us the healing promised in Scripture. We declare, by Jesus' wounds we are healed. Thank you for forgiving us and redeeming our lives from destruction. You renew our youth and the hopes and dreams of our youth. The life of Jesus is the light that shines within each of us, and the darkness cannot overcome Him. Thank You that You sent Your Son that we might have *abundant* life. Amen

Leader gives guidelines for next session:
- **Read Beth Webb's testimony in Appendix I and read Session 2 in preparation for next week.**

Journal

Write down your "hope moment." Thank God for it and record any impressions or feelings you have about it.

Journal your thoughts and feelings about being in this group with other women. Did God speak to you through the sharing of another about your own life and journey? If so, in what way?

Session Two

Hope – Reclaiming Your Identity and Dreams

Why are you cast down, O my soul? And why are you disquieted within me? Hope in God for I shall yet praise him who is the health of my countenance and my God. Psalm 43:5

The reality that I was going to lose control of my body, appearance, and ability to be of use to anyone began to set in. In this, God uncovered my core believe that I am only of value through my usefulness to others…I lay awake at night and tearfully asked God if the best part of my life was over and the bad (or the end) part was beginning. – Beth Webb

In a way, a diagnosis of breast cancer can traumatize our souls the way 9/11 traumatized America—we knew instinctively our world would never be the same! In the face of breast cancer and it's residual distress we may be surprised to discover thoughts we've carried about God, our bodies, and what makes us valuable. We may also encounter an unprecedented sense of loss and grief.

This session we'll look at that loss and grief regarding who we are as women. We'll consider our body image, our perceived destiny, hopes, and dreams, and how that has been diminished, transformed, and in some cases strengthened.

Seeing in the dark
Beth stated, "God uncovered my core belief that I am only of value through my usefulness to others." Below, several women share their personal revelations about how breast cancer changed their lives and understanding of themselves.

> *Prior to my diagnosis, I saw my purpose in life as being a woman of prayer (intercessor), healing minister and teacher, and an ambassador for Christ in the marketplace. I had a pretty good sense of purpose for the Lord and felt that what I was spending my time on was worthwhile and Kingdom-advancing. However, I became aware of an unhealthy self-sufficiency and independence that I could no longer utilize, if I was to come through my cancer treatment...*
>
> *Diagnosis caused me to have a very strong desire "to not lose a body part" in the course of my treatment. I just didn't want to be deformed. I like to swim and I did not want to look unattractive in my swimming suit. I do hope to remarry at some point and thought about not being attractive physically to my potential husband. ...The thought of living my life alone, and with a deformity, was very painful to consider.*
> – Anthonie

*I became aware of an
unhealthy self-sufficiency
and independence...*

Patterns of shame revealed

> *[After] My total mastectomy, one breast then the other two months later (due to discovering BRCA2), I felt like half a woman. I was so ashamed of my body that I showed every female in my family (cousins, sisters, daughter) how I looked. I acted kind of proud because I was so embarrassed. ... I made a joke of it, that's how I have always acted and gotten by.* – Cindy Martin

> *...I felt an incredible amount of shame that I had breast cancer. I felt that I had lost the favor of God, and that I must have done something wrong to cause this i.e. holding negative emotions in, stress and worry, past/current sin issues. Even to this day, I am cautious about chasing after "root issues" for breast cancer, etc., because it caused me a lot of guilt, shame and confusion. But I do know that God has used and is still using this cancer experience in my life to unveil deep heart pains, woundings and ungodly beliefs, and using it to bring me to a greater place of freedom and wholeness.* – Patti

There was a feeling of betrayal that something so deadly could have been growing quietly inside of me.

Inconsolable losses

At the time of the second diagnosis, my husband and I had just begun the process of adopting a six-year-old boy from China. We had been unofficially "matched" to this boy (our US adoption agency had his dossier waiting to officially match him to us). China was just changing their policies and we were encouraged to push ahead with this during my treatments by a friend, and try to get the doctors' medical information before the official diagnosis was released. We couldn't. We did not have the strength, stamina nor did it feel right to do so. We had to put this on hold until after all the chemo and radiation treatments were completed. After the treatments, the Chinese agency gave an emphatic "no" and demanded this little boy's dossier back. We were denied adoption and the Chinese government's guideline for qualification was a 10-year cancer-free history. We had to face the fact that we would probably not have children as the chemo and Arimidex treatments sent me into early menopause. – Patti

Chemo defined life as a "one day at a time" enterprise. I didn't indulge in any processing of sadness or anger about my condition. Being sad or angry wasn't

going to change that I had cancer. On the other hand, there was a feeling of betrayal that something so deadly could have been growing quietly inside of me, while I moved through life comparatively without cares. – Beth

Dreams that cry out for more of God

When I was a child growing up inside a large Chinese church in Manila, where my father was the pastor, my heart cried out to see God step out of the Bible and walk in power and authority. Now [with the advent of cancer] *the heart of that young girl dared Him to be such a God.* – Jean

Cancer is a magnifying glass: Hidden fears are exposed, our view of God and self sometimes become shockingly clearer. But in the mix, dreams and hopes are also shown in more precise and precious relief. Psalm 37:4 declares, "Take delight in the LORD, and he will give you the desires of your heart." Cancer can never change that.

Session 2: Hope—Reclaiming Your Identity and Dreams

Questions for Discussion & Reflection

- *"Time to Connect to Hope." Leader prays out loud, giving group members a moment to reflect:* **God, according to Your wisdom, remind us of a "hope" moment where You encouraged us about our losses, dreams, or body image in the face of breast cancer… or surface any other moment of hope in our lives where You demonstrated Your love.** *(pause). Leader continues,* **Let's take two to three minutes each to share what we saw, felt, or heard and why it inspires hope. If nothing surfaces, then share that. Take a moment to note what God surfaced for you in the Journal section.**

- We just read excerpts from other women about their responses to cancer, as well as shifts in perception regarding their purpose in life and view of self. Share how your experience with breast cancer has changed your perceived purpose, dreams of career, family, or ministry?

- What losses, are you grieving and where do you need God's comfort, restoration, and hope now?

Prayer
Leader prays out loud (as before) with participants repeating.

God, I thank You that Your Spirit is called the Comforter. I need Your comfort now. I give You my hopes, dreams, and plans, and ask You to revive or replace them with Your dreams for me. I know Your plans for me are good. I know

You will finish the work You've begun in me. I offer to You my greatest losses in the process of confronting this disease.

Leader asks them to speak their losses out loud to the group. Leader concludes prayer time with participants repeating

I know You are a God of restoration and resurrection. Restore my vision for life, resurrect my hope and heal my heart, mind, soul, and body. You have transported me from the kingdom of darkness into the kingdom of Your own Son—a kingdom full of light that eclipses all shadow.

Leader gives guidelines for next session:

- **Read and reflect on Session 3.**

- **Look through the list of Hope, Healing & Community Scriptures in Appendix II and pick one to meditate on.**

- **Also bring an object, poem, Scripture, picture, or article of clothing that had or has significant meaning or that brought hope into your cancer experience (from any phase: discovery, diagnosis, treatment, etc.).**

Leader brings closure to session by blessing the group and sealing all God has done.

Journal
Write down your "hope moment." Thank God for it and write down any impressions or feelings you have about it.

Journal your lost dreams or hopes. Ask the Father to show you the ones he is reviving and replacing. Write them down and thank Him for His redeeming love.

Session Three

Hope – Faith and Peace in Treatment Decisions

Do not be anxious about anything, but in every situation, by prayer and petition, with thanksgiving, present your requests to God. And the peace of God, which transcends all understanding, will guard your hearts and your minds in Christ Jesus. Philippians 4:6-7

I found out quickly that people have strong opinions on diagnostics and treatment of cancer. I was bombarded with phone calls from well-intended friends (and some people I didn't even know that well) urging me to not let "them" do any invasive procedure on me. I was overwhelmed at my lack of knowledge. Then I became irritated that I was becoming a case in point for their strongly held viewpoints and snapped at one such person: "This is happening to ME!" An important lesson for myself in freely giving advice.

From the first day the possibility of cancer was uttered, disagreement arose in my surrounding community about receiving treatment and surgery. Is chemo in reality the option that spiritual losers choose? The conflict was around having treatment or letting God heal me. People really got emotional about it. I knew what it felt like to receive that kind of faith, having seen God heal miraculously. However, again I heard that whisper that I was going to descend into this "valley of the shadow of death," yet I would know His presence there. God wouldn't let me go there without something redemptive in mind... Right? I also told myself that if God removed the cancer at the front end, I probably wouldn't appreciate it, because I have always been healthy—I would just get out of going through something hard. However, when confronted by the "go-for-the-healing" contingent, I felt some guilt for not having enough faith to not get treatment and surgery. Did Jesus have a disappointed look on His face too?

My former bosses and mentors, Andy and Jonathan, prayed for me, giving what turns out to have been the pivotal words. They said that God wasn't so concerned with me having enough faith to be healed, as entrusting myself to His goodness no matter what happens. Chemo wasn't a lack of faith, rather a means of waging war for my life. Andy prophesied that distilled through the suffering would be a joy and contentment with life. I felt great peace after those words. Indeed, going with the peace of the Lord, and not fear or guilt, became a refrain. The Lord would heal me—he would heal my wounds after surgery. My well-meaning, "faith-filled" friends calmed down after a while and got on board to stay. "Oh Lord, be the power that drives these drugs and the precision that guides the scalpel. Because here I go into that valley."— Beth Webb

Crying out for wisdom
Making decisions about our treatment, when faced with a life-altering condition may be one of the hardest things we'll ever do. The fear of making the wrong decision always looms. The insistent voices of well-meaning friends, family, doctors and pastors can add confusion to already difficult choices. When we look at the Bible there are many examples of sincere women and men of faith who faced hard decisions and even made wrong choices that didn't reflect obedience to God. One thing is clear; God is bigger than our choices.

> *God is divinely holy and sovereign. Right at the time of my diagnosis, I received a phone call from a prior mentor/friend whom I had not heard from in months and maybe even years. She felt the Lord led her to call me. She asked me what was happening. I told her. It turned out she had just gone through breast cancer herself! It ended up being similar in staging and lymph node activity as mine (microscopic). She shared how the Lord had spoken to her to "go natural." I remember in my mind thinking "Oh, Lord, I don't have the faith for that..."*
>
> *I remembered a book I received years before from a Christian doctor who shared that as he treated each patient, he asked the Lord for the "healing path" for that person. He mentioned each healing path might be different. This released me to follow what I felt in my heart was right for me. I did feel the conventional means was what I was comfortable with. I chose to follow the doctors' recommendations. – Patti*

Concerned but not helpful

> *Four doctors told me I would die if I did not hurry to get chemo and radiation. My oncologist pointedly said to me, "We are fighting for your life. What other options do you have besides what we can do for you?" I wanted to say to them, "I do have the most powerful option. It is my faith in the God who heals." But I did not say anything. I know all rationale stops there at the edge of their medical knowledge. It is all about their medical knowledge.*
>
> *Yet when I try to work with their reports, I find them to be confusing and having no solutions for true healing. Proverbs 3 says we are to acknowledge Him in all our ways, and He will direct our path. When I consider cancer treatments without the possibility of God in the picture, it brings death, not peace and life to my spirit.*
>
> *Nevertheless, I received a good word from a prayer friend that God would be with me if I choose to go into treatments and He would be with me if I believe I am miraculously healed and no longer need to go into treatments. My final choice—in regards to what I felt was God's leading—was the latter.* – Jean

The blessing and burden of choice

> *From the very beginning my faith and desired hope was to be supernaturally healed. I prayed and asked for prayer from everybody that believed in divine healing. I thought God was going to zap me and heal me instantly in a supernatural way. I had such a high level of faith and expectancy for a supernatural*

healing. And this is when my boat sunk—I don't know a better expression to state what I felt. I continued with doctor's appointments and more tests hoping to hear from somebody, "You don't have any more cancer." Nobody said it. I was so very disappointed. The surgeon talked to me about different possible dates for surgery. I didn't give her an answer for a couple of weeks. I finally said to myself, "OK — surgery and six weeks of radiation." Surgery felt like the right decision and finally I had peace with it. I heard the Lord tell me, "Surgery is one way I heal." The other phrase I heard is, "You are going to be okay." I so wanted to move forward with my life and put cancer behind me.

After those six weeks, the oncologist recommended that I take a certain medication for five years; it consisted of one pill a day every day. I researched it thoroughly; didn't like the side effects, went to see another doctor for a second opinion. He said pretty much the same thing, just changing the name of the pill. So, after a lot of prayer and research and receiving peace with my decision, I never took the prescriptions and never went back to see the oncologists. – Hadassah

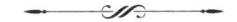

> Oh Lord, be the power that
> drives these drugs and the
> precision that guides the
> scalpel. Because here I go
> into that valley.

I never felt that "chemo was the option spiritual losers choose," but it was not helpful during the time of treatment when people would say that I was putting "poison" in my system and that chemo drugs could cause cancer in themselves. It may have been true, but it was not helpful because it just fed into the fear and helplessness. I just prayed God's covering over me – it was all I could do.

Later, different people approached me about different prayer models, about different dietary supplements, etc., but it was too much and it was too confusing. – Patti

Peace...and war

I did experience the peace of God in my treatment decisions. I had such a profound sense of the Lord's peace that kept me moving forward as I had four chemo treatments and then moved on to radiation for six weeks. The chemo was really tough emotionally, and I hit a place where I felt really unstable and out of control, and that was terrifying. – Anthonie

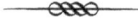

While I was going back and forth about what God wanted me to do about the medical treatments, I was surprised to hear Him ask me, "What do you want out of this?" Without any thinking, my heart said, "I want to experience miraculous healing."

My spirit cried out to Him, "You have to deliver me from cancer. You have to heal me completely. God, Send troops into my body to fight against the cancerous cells and help my good cells to win. I have traveled this far with You, climbing high mountains and walking through many valleys of the shadow of death with You holding my hand. It is time I know you as Jehovah Rapha, the God who heals." – Jean

Abiding love
Despite the confusion, whatever decisions we embrace, whether natural, surgical, chemical, or a combination of select options, the good news is we're never alone in our treatment journey. As we respond to His invitation for relationship, God stays with us through all of our choices, redirects us when necessary, and shelters us with His love. We can be certain when we make Christ our savior and sanctuary He never leaves us or forsakes us…ever.

Session 3: Hope–Faith and Peace in Treatment Decisions

Questions for Discussion & Reflection

- "Time to Connect to Hope." *Participants each share about the objects (last week's assignment) they have brought and why they are significant. Afterward, Leader prays out loud giving group members a moment to reflect:* **God, according to Your wisdom, remind us of a "hope" moment in the process of making decisions about our treatment ... or surface any other moment of hope in our lives where You demonstrated Your love.** *(pause). Leader continues,* **Let's take two to three minutes each to share what we saw, felt, or heard and why it inspires hope. If nothing surfaces, then share that. Take a moment to note what God surfaced for you in the Journal section.**

- At what stage are you in making treatment decisions?

- How have doctors, friends, and/or Scriptures added to your faith... or created confusion about treatment choices?

- How much of God's peace are you experiencing (or did you experience) in your treatment decisions? What feels settled and what feels uncertain?

Prayer
Leader instructs the group to break into pairs. Have each person, in turn, share with their partner their hopes and concerns regarding treatment decisions. The other prayer partner simply listens and responds by blessing them with God's clarity and peace in decision-making.

Allow 10 minutes for the preceding time of sharing and blessing.

Leader continues prayer time out loud with participants repeating.

Thank You Lord, that You are bigger than my confusion. You are greater than my fear, questions or uncertainty. Thank You that whatever treatment decisions we make, You are here with us, shepherding us through. Quiet competing voices, so that we may hear You when *You* speak. Give us confidence in our own response to Your leading. Though we walk through the valley of the shadow of death, we will fear no evil, for You are always and ever with us. Surely goodness and mercy will follow us all the days of our life and we will dwell in Your house Lord forever (Psalm 23, paraphrase).

Leader brings closure to session by blessing the group and sealing all God has done.

Journal
Write down your "hope moment." Thank God for it and note any impressions or feelings about it.

Reflect on Philippians 4:6-7 (the Scripture noted at the beginning of this chapter). Write down any impressions or results from your prayer time.

Session Four

Hope – Inviting Jesus into Your Weakness

But he said to me, "My grace is sufficient for you, for my power is made perfect in weakness." Therefore I will boast all the more gladly about my weaknesses, so that Christ's power may rest on me. 2 Corinthians 12:9

In prayer we need to speak whatever truth is in us; pain and grief, fear and disappointment, yearning and desire, questions and doubt, hope and faith, failure and weakness, praise and thanks, despair and sorrow, anger, and yes, even hatred. – Marjorie J. Thompson (as quoted in Beth Webb's testimony)

As women, we sometimes hear different messages about who we are and how we should experience things, behave, or respond. But we are manifold in our makeup and temperament. Being willing to allow Christ into our weakness, at its core, is about being able to set aside the ways we've been named by others. Then we are able to let go of the expectations we and those around us have for our lives and hear the voice of the Father.

Each of us is as different as the women we read about in the Bible. And words like weak, strong, emotion, courage, tears, or "getting real" evoke different images and emotions from each of us. There are those of us for whom anger is strictly off limits, and for others it is the "go-to" emotion. Some of us have made inner vows, by example, "I will not cry," while others are comfortable with a wide range of emotions, both internally and visibly.

Encountering cancer, we find it's a dangerous world. However we respond, and whoever we are, God wants to meet us in the midst of our pain—masks off, wounds exposed. We work so hard at trying to hide our weaknesses from other people that we often do the same with God. When we are under pressure, tired, sick, overwhelmed, sometimes a person emerges that is a "stranger" to us. We even hide from ourselves. As Debbie Driscoll, associate director of Embracing Life Ministries, says, "You've got to get to know that stranger, baby!" But be encouraged, though our responses sometime surprise us, they never ever surprise God.

I chose to turn my face towards God, even when I didn't feel His presence.

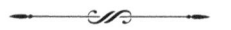

Getting real with God
Sometimes we feel like we need to clean up, appear stronger, more holy or forgiving than we are. We might declare God's Word one day with confidence and faith over our illness; the next we are spouting Scriptures frantically to appear in control or to gain God's approval. Thankfully, we can rest in Him no matter what. God's love, saving grace and mercy is greater than our biggest mistake, our worst attitude, or our deepest despair.

Beth, in her story (Appendix I) has expressed that in her journey with God toward healing, she realized what hadn't been formed in her was living with "uncertainty and the value of weakness." Although Beth was assured of God's faithfulness, for her there was a terrible suspense in not knowing exactly how long this fragility/weakness might last. What real "value" or purpose could be mined from this unexpected detour? Like most of us, Beth did not want to spend a second longer than necessary in the place of shadows.

Although some have said their sickness "has been a gift"—the sickness isn't from God! "God works all things to the good for those who love him and are called according to his purposes" (Rom 8:28). All things are not good, but Jesus will get every bit of positive mileage out of every situation. That's His job. He's the Redeemer. It's hard for us to grasp that although God did not "strike" us with illness, He still does some of His most profound healing and deliverance in the midst of suffering and persecution. And He is powerfully present.

Weakness and suffering had little place in my spirituality prior to being treated for cancer. When I had meditated on the humanity of Jesus, I had never thought of Him getting sick or injured. He had a job to do and, without consideration, I assumed God had kept Him from physical affliction until the passion. (And I went through all my systematic theology classes assuming that!) I had seen suffering as the result of sin, or an "educational occasion." Aside from the pain of the woundings of my soul that I sought healing for, times of suffering were more like a test to be passed, shed, and moved on from. However, entering into a suffering that I couldn't shed changed those assumptions and how I related to God.

Vineyard pastor John Wimber (who also had cancer) said about walking through the valley of the shadow of death: "...it's frightening. Its uncertainties keep you alert to every changing scenario." The threat of the unknown can be overwhelming. I had to embrace the truth that I could not control or plan my life. God is accomplishing His work in me, even through suffering. He is my peace. – Beth

Jesus will get every bit of positive mileage out of every situation. That's His job. He's the Redeemer

I need HELP!!!!
Life doesn't stop when we get cancer: Jobs don't end, families need to be cared for, and bills must be paid. But sometimes we are too weak to do the simplest of tasks. Cancer doesn't stop God's abundant and transforming life either. He will meet us in the middle of our neediness with both power and intimacy, even when we can't, won't, or don't want to recognize it. Sometimes the way he meets us is through supernatural provision of strength, or resources— human and/or financial—but just as often he does it through community. That may require acknowledging our need and seeking help (more about this in Session 6). Sometimes we just have to ask someone to help us find help.

I was in denial until I was having my second chemo treatment and had an emotional meltdown while sitting in the chair. All of a sudden, I felt anger, which really surprised me. Where had that come from? It

> was at this time that I made the decision to take an anti-depressant and seek personal therapy. I had a flood of memories to process at this point. It took me a while to come to terms with the fact that managing my emotions in this way was not a "wimpy decision," but rather, a really healthy self-care decision. This was because I had been so self-sufficient for so many years of my life.
>
> It took me over a year after radiation ended to begin to process the grief. The vulnerability and weakness were much easier to accept. The grief felt different and was harder to manage, though I tried with the anti-depressant (that I went on and off of a few times). Finally, however, I was strong enough emotionally and physically to allow myself to feel my grief and ditch the anti-depressant.–Anthonie

Meeting God in the shadows

It takes a different kind of strength to allow oneself to experience the weakness of grief, the pain of loss and be willing to meet Christ there.

> It was a shock to have a diagnosis again. I had passed the five-year mark, but realized that it was no comfort as I discovered cancer could hit anytime. I did recognize that I had not addressed certain issues the first time and that they were left unresolved. One major issue was my loss of trust in the Lord, especially in His protection over me. I had to also deal with any residual anger towards the Lord. I had to deal with the fear/panic attacks that had surfaced so strongly during that first time and had never left.

This time, I honestly grieved more. I chose to turn my face towards God, even when I didn't feel His presence and especially when I felt so ashamed of my negative feelings towards Him. I had to hold onto to the belief that He was big enough to take my anger and any other surprising—to me—emotions that came up. He was not surprised. He was not unaware or without understanding. – Patti

In our weakness, the strength of Jesus is a banner of love over our fear.

When fear engulfed me and my mind seemed frozen, I reached out to Jesus and heard Him say to me: "Come to Me, all you who are split up. Come to Me, and Let Me love you into wholeness and oneness. I have come to fight cancer. I have come to give life and life abundant. Speak that to your own body, Jean, and to your good cells. I live inside you. You have my power to speak life to your own cells. Do it." – Jean

Session 4: Hope–Inviting God into Your Weakness

Questions for Discussion & Reflection

- *"Time to Connect to Hope." Leader prays out loud, giving group members a moment to reflect:* **Father, according to Your wisdom, remind us of a "hope" moment where Jesus met us in our weakness with His strength, or the Holy Spirit came with needed comfort … or surface any other moment of hope in our lives where You demonstrated Your love.** *(pause). Leader continues,* **Let's take two to three minutes each to share what we saw, felt, or heard and why it inspires hope. If nothing surfaces, then share that. Take a moment to note what God surfaced for you in the Journal section.**

- When you hear the words "living with uncertainty," what feelings and thoughts come up for you? Describe how you deal with the uncertainty and weakness you experience?

- When you find yourself "in the valley," in what ways do you experience God being with you? If you don't, describe what that's like.

- Is it easy or scary to share your weakness and needs? (With people?) (With God?) In what ways would you like to be able to ask for help?

- "He Himself took our weaknesses and carried our diseases." (Mt. 8:17, Holman Bible).
    o In what ways, if any, has the meaning of this Scripture changed for you?

Prayer
Break up into twos share any areas of weakness and vulnerability that you desire prayer from your partner about: physical, spiritual, emotional. Take turns praying for each other (total time 10 minutes).

Leader gives guidelines for next session

Read and reflect on Session 5. Look through the list of Hope, Healing & Community Scriptures in Appendix II and pick one to meditate on and bring next week to share in our discussion time.

Leader closes with a short prayer of blessing

Thank You Father that Your grace sustains us and that Your power is perfected in weakness. We confess we are weak, but You are strong. We pray for joy, and hope, and that out of Your glorious riches You will strengthen us with power through Your Spirit in our inner being. We declare that the same power that raised Christ from the dead is able to resurrect our physical bodies. Revive us again, that we may rejoice in You now and forever. In Jesus name Amen. (Paraphrase of Ephesians 3:16, 1:19-20; and Romans 8:11.)

Journal
Offer your weakness to God and ask Him to replace it with His strength. Ask what He wants to give you and write down any impressions or feelings you may have. Bless and thank Him.

Session Five

Hope – Emerging from the Shadow of Breast Cancer (Prayer)

Now to him who is able to do immeasurably more than all we ask or imagine, according to his power that is at work within us, to him be glory in the church and in Christ Jesus throughout all generations, for ever and ever! Amen. Ephesians 3:20-21

At the lowest points, vision was shrunk down to what my body felt like and was doing (or not doing). I wondered if my life was going to be anything more than a fuzzy brain, aching joints, feeling psycho with steroids, and a turtle-like appearance. There was one clear vertical experience with the Lord. Waking one morning I received what I believe was a word from Him. It wasn't a Scripture, worship song, words from St. John of the Cross, Mother Teresa, [Dietrich] Bonhoeffer, [Henry] Nouwen, or a friend. I was encouraged by the words of James Bond in the book Dr. No, *spoken after he had survived a diabolical obstacle course designed, by Dr. No, to kill him in several different ways.*

> All he needed was an ounce of hope, an ounce of reassurance that it was still worthwhile trying to stay alive... On an instinct he felt his pulse. It was slow, but regular. The steady thump of life revived his spirits. What the hell was he worrying about? He was alive. The wounds and bruises on his body were nothing—absolutely nothing. They looked ugly, but nothing was broken. Inside the torn envelope, the machine was quietly, solidly ticking over... Get moving! Clean yourself and wake up! *(Fleming, 205)*

There may be poison and a cocktail of drugs in my system. I may be hairless and have a puffy moon face. But my heart was still beating like it should. I could still walk, talk, and tell you who I was. I could tell you who you were, and where I was going. Overall, I was okay, good to go. The Lord had given some lighthearted perspective. – Beth Webb

Relationship at the core of all healing

Our relationship with Christ is the cornerstone of our healing. Many of us have thought, "If I work hard enough, I might get rewarded with a "healing." Yet, it's really all about His sacrifice on the Cross and our simple act of surrender to His love. The enemy of our souls would love us to think of God as someone who we manipulate into doling out presents by offering sacrifices, by doing the "right" things: reading the Bible, praying, contemplating, listening, declaring. If we put together the right formula, we might just hit the healing jackpot! But that would make healing all about us. Reading the Bible, prayer, confession, and repentance are all good and necessary for our healing and transformation. However, they are part of the rhythm of a loving relationship, not coins in a healing slot machine.

God's intentions are already those of healing and restoration. One of His names is *Jehovah Rapha*, the Lord who heals us. It is the Father's good pleasure to give us the kingdom, which includes all manner of healing.

People healed in the Bible sometimes made great efforts to get to where Jesus was. Even now, we all yearn to be taken to where Jesus is, forgetting that by His spirit He is always near; in fact if we have made Him Lord, He is in us. Beth's journey through the shadows, as she dealt with the ravages of chemo, robbed her of the strength to win God's attention through spiritual activity.

> *After the early days following diagnosis, I had no vertical experience of the Lord's presence—no amazing prayer times or visions. During treatment, I can count on one hand how many times I opened my Bible. The disciplines cited earlier [*Scripture reading, Lectio Divina, listening prayer, etc.*] were absent.* – Beth

Let go and receive
Even had she wanted to, Beth could not have *earned* her healing by spiritual "activity." Let's release ourselves from performance-driven faith, and learn to rest in the finished work of the Cross.

> *About a year after the diagnosis and having just completed my treatments a few months before, I was at Mammoth Lakes. One night, I couldn't sleep and went out on the balcony and looked at the incredible sky above with its unending vastness of stars. I remember crying out to the Lord, "Where are You?" I felt He had*

abandoned me. As I gazed at the sky, wanting some answer, my eyes caught a star twinkling in and out of my eyesight – in view, then blinking out of view for seconds, and then blinking back into view again. In that moment, I felt like the Spirit spoke to my spirit that God is like this. Just because I didn't see Him or feel His presence, He was still there. He didn't leave. He hadn't moved. He was still there, though I couldn't perceive His presence. He was faithful. That night was a significant personal breakthrough for me on this journey. – Patti

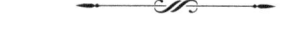

I felt He was giving me a choice and I chose to live...

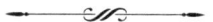

My life just took one huge shift through this process of cancer treatment. I decided that I wanted to live after taking two days or so to go deep with the Lord about wanting to live or die. I felt He was giving me a choice and I chose to live. I just had such a strong awareness of His desire for me to live...that there were things He had for me to do with my life. In all the years of my life when I really did want to "go home and be with the Lord," I finally came to see that living was what He really wanted of me. I don't allow myself to go to that place in my emotions anymore where I just want to die because life is too hard. Now, I feel the Lord's presence with me so strongly. I am doing life with the Trinity now and feel integrated and whole spiritually, emotionally, and physically, not to mention relationally which has been such a huge breakthrough for me. I do

feel loneliness at times, but now can reach out to others. – Anthonie

Session 5: Hope–Emerging from the Shadow of Breast Cancer (Prayer)

Questions for Discussion & Reflection

- *"Time to Connect to Hope." Leader prays out loud, giving group members a moment to reflect:* **Father, according to Your wisdom, remind us of a moment where You revealed Yourself or Your love to us… or surface any moment of hope or encouragement in our lives.** *(pause). Leader continues,* **Let's take two to three minutes each to share what we saw, felt, or heard and why it inspires hope. If nothing surfaces, then share that. Take a moment to note what God surfaced for you in the Journal section.**

- Share the Scripture you picked from Appendix II and describe why you selected it.

Prayer (*for emergence from the shadow of breast cancer*)
Leader prays as before in short phrases with participants repeating.

✝ **Heavenly Father, Lord Jesus Christ and Holy Spirit, we come boldly before Your throne, with our sisters in Christ as witnesses, in the knowledge that we are blessed with every spiritual blessing in Christ. We proclaim the living hope that we can do all things through Christ who strengthens us. It is with this certainty that we offer these prayers of faith.**

✝ **We give thanks for Your redeeming and healing love, for Your good plans for us, for Your promise to never leave us or forsake us. We declare that Your mercy and love are greater: greater than sickness, greater than** judgment, greater than cancer. We thank you for the free unearned gifts of salvation and healing.

☩ Together, we bring before You all the fearful, destructive feelings, thoughts, and false imaginations that have attached themselves to our diagnosis of breast cancer. We renounce any lies that "raise themselves up against the knowledge of God." We proclaim we are in no way being punished or disciplined by You with this cancer. You will *redeem* this experience to Your glory. Forgive us for accepting a distorted view of who You are and how You care for Your children.

☩ By Your power and through Your name, we declare You give us love for fear… and hope for despair and devastation. We take hold of Your revelation of our womanhood; You call us beautiful. We renounce and turn away from words we have knowingly or unknowingly allowed to name and shape us, such as unwanted, unlovely, undesirable, helpless, hopeless, or worthless.

☩ We honor You for sending Your only begotten Son, Jesus Christ, for our salvation, healing and transformation: He has borne our sicknesses and by His wounds we are healed!

☩ Your presence in us, Holy Spirit, is our assurance of eternal hope and life.

☩ Lord, we ask You now to let Your kingdom come and Your will be done in our bodies.

☩ As sisters in Christ, united in our holy bond of hope, help us encourage one another and others facing a similar diagnosis. Together, through Jesus Christ our Lord,

we *will* overcome this adversity, giving glory to You, our Heavenly and Loving Father.   Amen.

Journal
Talk to God about your hope moment and write down any additional words or impressions. Thank him.

Ask God to show what He is accomplishing in you through prayer and the community of this group. Write down your impressions.

Session Six

Hope – Embracing God's Community of Healing (Testimonies)

For just as each of us has one body with many members, and these members do not all have the same function, so in Christ we, though many, form one body, and each member belongs to all the others.
Romans 12:4-5

I feared being a burden and, in turn, being rejected. I tried to push people away at the beginning. I gave them an out, warning them this wasn't going to be pleasant. I was not going to be able to be present, probably a self-absorbed bore. I would understand if they wanted to reconsider the commitment they made to walk with me. To the person, they listened politely and told me to knock it off. What this really was, of course, was the fear of being known in weakness. In reality, I loathed my weakness, believing it to be repellant. This also uncovered a disregard I had probably always had for other's vulnerability. On reflection, I see that God was working on another kind of miracle—revealing His love for me through my family of faith, right in the center of what I feared most. He was going to heal me of more than wounds from surgery.

Nobody left me. They seemed to have endless kindness, comfort, and ability to be present—God's voice, face, arms and hands. I had to sit there and take it without anything to give in return. That is hard for me. Being weak and nevertheless cared for exposed my quest up to that point, to be respected and admired, over being known and loved. – Beth Webb

Belonging involves risk
Jesus is our example. Though He withdrew sometimes to solitary places, for rest and communion with His Father, He lived out His life in community. He showed us clearly that His kingdom was based on mutual care, love, encouragement, celebration and—never to be overlooked—shared grief and lament. Community is not always easy to find, or easy to be part of. Our reservations about the church body, however, may rob us of God's good gift of community. As Psalm 68 says, "God sets the lonely in families, he leads out the prisoners with singing" (v.6a).

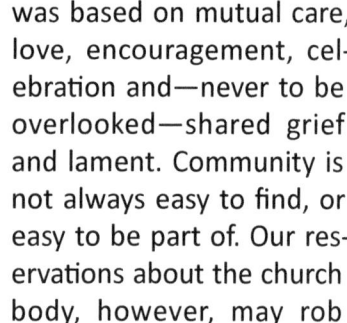

Love the others that I love... Know that when you are weak they will be your strength.

Healing is a lifelong process and will take place in many contexts, with many different people, and via an assortment of means and relationships. To embrace healing is to embrace God and His healing community.

I grew up with the fear of people and had a nervous breakdown when I was working on my master's thesis in California. Towards the end of my year of fighting breast cancer, I wrote in my journal that I was beginning to see myself as a part of the bride of Christ, not as people who could hurt me, but as a part of who I was. In my spirit I heard Him say, "Love the others that I love. They are a part of you and you are a part of them. Know that when you are weak they will be your strength. When your faith is low, their strong faith in Me will hold you up." – **Jean**

One Healer, many contexts

Once again, I went into a quieter place. During treatments, I stayed fairly quiet but close friends stayed by my side through prayer. I was back at my prior church after my marriage and I felt the loving support of the Body there. I attended a local church closer to home, and the Lord ministered to me there through worship, messages, and prayer ministers. I also attended art therapy again, allowing the Lord to use that to surface areas of emotional difficulty.

After treatments, I attended the Embracing Life Series *for the first time. This was such a pivotal ministry for me to attend. This was finally the "Christian" setting I was longing for where I could share all my questions, confusion, and struggles without judgment, criticism or even raising guilt-ridden concern from loved ones. Also, at the same time, the Lord gave opportunity to begin flag worship twice monthly in our church sanctuary with a few friends. This was also a significant time of worship before God, releasing that part of me to just "be," to grieve, release my pain and commune with*

God in the midst of this painful season. I also received deep healing prayer through Restoring the Foundations Ministry—powerful and realigning. I also attended a two-year spiritual direction program and part of this gem was having a spiritual director where I could continue to process and deal with the uncertainty of cancer. I continue meeting with her to this day. It has been an invaluable gift from God. I am learning to stay centered in the Lord, and to be honest before God and keep my face turned towards Him. –Patti

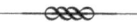

New vision brings more life

There have been two main shifts during the last year, bringing overall widening and deepening within my spiritual life: One has been the focus on community; God relating to me through the people walking with me, and me allowing it to happen. Following that shift was a deeper reckoning with weakness, giving place to suffering in the process of transformation... In relationships, the role I played was of helper/servant, rarely the one receiving. However, illness overturned that dynamic. My union with Christ was through my companions. In my spiritual life, the role of the body of Christ had not been as opened up as it is now. Surrendering to a season of receiving has brought more rest to my spiritual life. –Beth

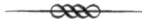

Regarding hope-filled input from the Lord or friends, well they all tell me the Lord is going to use my journey for His glory, and I agree. I just feel different now. It's difficult to describe how I feel, but I think

it's just that I live in the moment instead of the past or the future. I now welcome those the Lord brings across my path; the walls of self-sufficiency and independence are really gone. I am thankful when I can help others. The Lord is showing me that He wants to use me even when I can't see it. He recently told me that I mattered to Him and that just made my day! – Anthonie

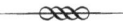

The cancer journey allowed me to appreciate and embrace the different parts of the expression of Christ. Since my cancer diagnosis, especially after the second time, I have been discovering and rediscovering the "being" part of me, the part of me that just loves to be in the presence of the Lord, communing, worshipping and praying as He leads. In this I find my greatest source of strength, delight and joy and I am discovering great freedom in that. I rediscovered the sacrifice of worship in this place of pain. This time also uncovered so much performance and approval-based service done on the outside while the inside was lifeless or dying. – Patti

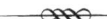

My self-sufficiency was fierce, due to early life neglect that caused me to come to the conclusion that no one was going to take care of me, so I would have to do it myself; that was how I lived my life up to the point of the cancer diagnosis. My priorities have changed in a big way. The Lord showed me all the striving I had engaged in for approval and acceptance, and that that was not what He was requiring of me. I have a lot more compassion and humility now in those places where pride had previously been. – Anthonie

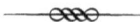

I am learning to say "NO" to all intimidations that make me submit to cancer as my lot. What God is after is for my spirit to emerge gloriously powerful and full of light. – Jean

Hope realized…for today and tomorrow

I always felt my relationship with God was like a lottery—maybe he will answer me today, if he's not too busy. My relationship with the Lord is very close now. I know he hears and knows my voice. I know the Bible says that he does, but reading and knowing is very different. I don't feel I have to prove to anyone my relationship with God. I know I'm His daughter and when I call Him, He always hears me and loves me. – Cindy

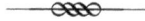

Finally, I don't believe that God planned for me to get cancer as part of a scripted drama or that my affliction had some purpose in itself; it only has meaning as it is redeemed by Christ on the Cross. Things are a complex web of circumstances with many agents playing a role. God did not miraculously intervene and deliver me from the journey, and I'll never know why. He delivers us from evil, but not from going through the "shadow of death." Still, I arrive today trusting he is powerfully present within me and through others when I suffer and walk through that valley. He suffers with me as he did during His life, in Gethsemane and on the Cross. The power of His presence within and without will "restore my soul" and uphold me as I continue to walk in uncertainty and grief. – Beth

I don't know if I have any conclusions, but I have many "learnings." I am learning to trust in God's Goodness. I am learning to let go of control and surrender and trust the One who does have control. I may not fully understand everything and why I had to go through cancer—not just once, but twice. I am learning that God is indeed sovereign. I don't know why we couldn't adopt a boy when he was six years old, but we marvel at the miraculous hand of God in opening the door six years later when we had let go of ever having any family. Now, that very boy is our son! I am learning to trust in His Voice that leads. I am learning that I can embrace life on a so much deeper level than what is seen on the human level of suffering from cancer—not to negate the suffering and pain, but that we can have a life in the Spirit that transcends this life on earth. We can hold onto and embrace that spiritual and eternal life that is within us through Christ our Lord. That is the more abundant life. I am learning to walk in the truths of God. – Patti

We live in a fallen, broken world filled with disease and strife. Sometimes it feels as if God has abandoned us. These are the times that test our faith. Do we let our circumstances sway our beliefs, or do we keep our eyes focused on our one true hope? Jesus. He never leaves us or forsakes us. He doesn't spare us from trials or the bad things this world has to offer, but he is always with us. Trials serve as the highlighter of our need for God. In and of ourselves we are limited. God is limitless. He has vast resources but his most valuable resources are you and me. – Terry

Hope Redeemed
Each day is filled with uncertainty. When we confront the shadowlands of breast cancer, we find that the control we may have thought we had over our lives is illusory. In facing a life-altering condition we come face-to-face with our own weakness. Fortunately we also discover Christ's healing power and the certainties of the Word and the redemption of our entire lives at the Cross. Hope is built and sustained as we rehearse those certainties, meditating on them, embracing them while staying connected to God and community. Christ will resurrect the kind of faith that gives substance, life and reality to our most expansive and glorious dreams and our deepest and most God-birthed hopes.

Session 6: Hope – Embracing God's Community of Healing

Questions for Discussion & Reflection

- "Time to Connect to Hope." *Leader prays out loud giving group members a time to reflect:* **Father, remind us of any shifts in perspective or words of encouragement that have arisen in the wake of last week's prayer.** *(pause). Leader continues,* **Let's take two to three minutes each to share what came up for each of us. Take a moment to note what God surfaced for you in the Journal section.**

- How has your experience with breast cancer changed the way you handle other difficult things in your life?

- How have you been impacted by this group? (In the areas of identity, faith and treatment, inviting God into your weakness, healing prayer, living in community?)

Prayer
Seal the time by praying out loud together.

To You who are able to keep us from falling and to present us before Your glorious presence without fault and with great joy—to the only God our Savior be glory, majesty, power and authority, through Jesus Christ our Lord, before all ages, now and forevermore! Amen (Jude 1:24-25, paraphrase).

Leader, in concluding More Hope!, encourages participants to utilize helpful resources in the Appendices, then closes with a prayer and blessing.

Journal
Reflect on and write down what you feel God has accomplished during our time together. Ask God to show you what is next in your healing journey. Offer him your questions and journal any impressions or feelings.

Appendix I

Journey of Hope: Beth Webb's Story

Prologue

November: Telling my story
The whole of the last twelve months, my life has been absorbed into a journey not of my choosing: the diagnosis and treatment for breast cancer that had spread into my lymph nodes. Almost all activities, including studies in seminary were suspended and redirected toward survival: five months of aggressive chemotherapy followed by surgery, followed by more chemotherapy, followed by radiation, and finally (if all goes well) follow-up anti-hormone therapy. My life has been forever changed by the journey. There is no going back to the way things were before. In fact, it's hard to recall what life was like before cancer. There have been irretrievable losses that I am grieving, as well as dividends I never could have foreseen.

Pre-cancer Background

Transformed by relationship
Marjorie J. Thompson, a writer and educator in the area of spiritual formation, focuses the general definition of "spirituality" on relationship: "God's way of relating to us, and our way of responding to God." Going further, Christian spirituality involves the "magnificent choreography of the Holy Spirit in the human spirit, moving us toward communion with both Creator and creation." It is both our capacity for this communion, as well as, how we flesh it out with life choices and practices. She refers to spiritual formation as the "reshaping according to the pattern we were created to bear," as Christ is formed in us (Gal. 4:19) recovering God's likeness, our true selves. (Thompson, *Soulfeast: An Invitation to the Christian Spiritual Life*, 6-7).

After coming back into the Christian faith in my late twenties, my life in the spirit has been geared toward experiencing and seeing transformation or change—the restoration of the *imago Dei* in me, which in time translated into ministry to others. The importance of change emanated from my ongoing struggle with relational brokenness and sexual addiction. Even as a Christian that dearly loved and desired to follow Christ, I wasn't able to walk in freedom and didn't know why. I had trouble apprehending God's presence, scant knowledge of who I was, and monumental insecurity. There didn't seem to be a solid center from which to make righteous choices. I needed healing. Therefore, I also had a profound need to hear/discern the voice of the Lord, and to know what he felt about me. I also yearned to experience and see God's power surpassing that of the sins committed against me, and that I had committed, bringing me into the life I was created for.

What emerged in my life in the spirit were emphases on individual union with Christ—cultivating intimacy with

Him, and the empowerment of the Holy Spirit unto a life that revealed transformation. A truth that drives through the center of both emphases is that my spirituality, no matter what character it has, is all God's initiative. I responded to Him because of His loving initiative toward me.

Disciplined by love and communion
Key to the cultivation of intimacy with Jesus, have been some spiritual disciplines, most notably prayer and the meditative reading of Scripture. Other disciplines have also been practiced (fasting, confession, fellowship, service) but these two have played the biggest part in my own sense of union with Christ. The practice of prayer and Scripture-reading weren't the result of hearing a teaching or reading a book. Rather, they sprung from a profound need to commune with God with my senses in the midst of my brokenness. Silence and prayer are sometimes differentiated as disciplines. I have a difficult time seeing silence as anything but prayer. What initially surfaced was a season of grieving, a deep well of pain. Pain gradually receded, giving way to much needed quiet within, and then speaking. Henri Nouwen writes that productive words find their beginning in silence. True relationship with my Father came to life, learning to talk to Him with unrehearsed, unstudied frankness. In *Soulfeast*, Thompson writes: "In prayer we need to speak whatever truth is in us; pain and grief, fear and disappointment, yearning and desire, questions and doubt, hope and faith, failure and weakness, praise and thanks, despair and sorrow, anger, and yes, even hatred." This candor has to be developed and returned to again and again, but deepens relationship. Significant healing of wounding happened as a prayer life took shape, eventually moving into intercession. The discipline of spiritual reading, or the meditative reading of the Scriptures has also been vital. Latching onto that objective source of truth

through exercises like the *Lectio Divina* led me to "encounter the Reality beyond the words."

Learning with the family
Life in the spirit has also been filled out in relationship to the Body of Christ. The "streams" or traditions in the church I have associated with are also significant. The charismatic stream has been the context for much of my formation; imparted was a love of the church with the Spirit's anointing for the equipping of God's people. Feeding into the charismatic stream are tributaries of holiness, the contemplative; the centrality of the Cross in transformation, and "the steady gaze of the soul upon the God who loves us," as Richard Foster describes. In these streams, with inner healing and participating in healing ministry, particularly with Desert Stream Ministries and the Vineyard Church, I had an overall sense of being carried toward wholeness.

This has been a cursory summary of fifteen years of spiritual formation. The "reshaping" has mainly been directed toward change (inner healing) and movement forward. From idolater to worshipper, addict to one free of addiction, from death to life.

Needy to "strong"? Upon reflection, what hadn't been developed was living with uncertainty and the value of weakness. Oh, I knew I was broken and, therefore, weak, and God was faithful to rest on me with His power (2 Cor. 12:9). I have seen God's faithfulness in my brokenness and His power unto transformation. Yet weakness was in the end something to aspire beyond. Suffering and/or loss of control were in a valley I was, in truth, wanting to ascend out of and leave behind.

The Descent

"I felt a lump." I mentioned matter-of-factly to my friend Erin, driving her home from the airport following Thanksgiving holiday. I was as surprised as she was to hear myself say it." I quickly waved off her solemn concern and changed the subject. She didn't leave the car without being assured I was being examined by a doctor and she didn't mean maybe.

The next day I sat shell-shocked as my physician made a phone call to the breast clinic to get me in for an immediate ultrasound and biopsy. She was "highly concerned"—the lump was "huge." I watched and listened for some reprieve in her insistence. None—there was no room for delay. As I left and drove home, I felt like I was walking underwater, and everyone's voice felt garbled and far away.

I had never known God relating to me in physical weakness. Of all the things I had cried out to in my life none had involved my own health. I had always been "as healthy as a horse" as they say. I had never wondered about being otherwise. I couldn't believe this was becoming an issue and neither could my friends and family. "There is sure another explanation," we all initially said. However, when I checked in to "listen," I heard a whisper "to brace myself yet remember His faithfulness." That's as far as I could hear or see. "Just move to the next step," I told myself.

December 30. Biopsy
In the meantime, I found out quickly that people have strong opinions on diagnostics and treatment of cancer. I was bombarded with phone calls from well-intended friends (and some people I didn't even know that well) urging me to not let "them" do any invasive procedure on me. I was overwhelmed at my lack of knowledge. Then I became irritated that I was becoming a case in point for their strongly held viewpoints and snapped at one such person: "This is

happening to ME!" An important lesson for myself in freely giving advice.

However, I indeed ended up delaying a month, pursuing a non-invasive diagnostic (which involved my hands being in icy water for several minutes while they took a reading of "hot" areas in my body) only for that person to tell me I had a "sick breast" and needed to get a biopsy right away. Enough already! Let's get on with this! So three weeks later, I found myself in a another surreal environ, lying on my side with my left arm above my head as a doctor and nurse shot a large needle into my breast removing tissue. The radiologist looked at me and spoke with a somber carefulness I was beginning to recognize. It looked like there were four tumors and the lymph nodes were looking suspicious. I was to call after New Year for the results but he would work on authorizing me to see a surgeon.

My dear friend and housemate, Donna, drove me home. Pasadena was filling up with college football fans for the Rose Bowl. My beloved Oklahoma Sooners were playing on New Year's Day. Before this cancer thing had entered my world I would have been happily anticipating game day, making chili, even trying to get a ticket. Looking out the window, I realized I had totally forgotten it was happening. I saw several people walking down the street decked out in their crimson and cream regalia. Fearing life with simple joys was receding quickly, I impulsively lowered the window and yelled out: "BOOMER SOONER!!" The fans returned the cry. Donna regarded me sideways. I went underwater again.

New Years went by as usual, going out with my closest friends. Everyone was caring, present, and committed to prayer for me. My Christian family was not going to take this lying down! However, I lay awake at night and tearfully asked God if the best part of my life was over and the bad (or the end) part was beginning. I don't do sick! This cannot be happening! I sensed an abyss nearby to slide into, although more so the Lord's presence—undoubtedly the result of the prayer going on.

Diagnosis

January 2. Worst fears realized
I closed the door to my office at work and received the call from the radiologist who performed the biopsy. He confirmed that the tumors in my left breast were malignant. More scans and biopsies were needed to see if it had spread to the lymph nodes.

A couple of days later, accompanied by my great friends Gwen and Erin, I sat in the surgeons office who laid out for me what he and the oncologist were going to do to get rid of the cancer. It would involve ten months if all went as expected. I would begin with chemotherapy to shrink the tumors, then surgery, then radiation. I would lose all my hair (temporarily) and a quarter of my left breast. It looked like the tumors were localized in the bottom left quadrant of my left breast which was better than them being spread out. It was a relief to hear someone say what they were going to DO about the problem—not just tell me I had one. The surgeon also gave me the option of doing a double mastectomy and reconstruction of the breasts. I chose to try and save the breast and told Dr. Faddis to fire the whole arsenal at the damned thing.

Impossible Decisions

Is chemo in reality the option spiritual losers choose?
From the first day the possibility of cancer was uttered, disagreement arose in my surrounding community about receiving treatment and surgery. *Is chemo in reality the option spiritual losers choose?* The conflict was around having treatment or letting God heal me. People really got emotional about it. I knew what it felt like to receive that kind of faith,

having seen God heal miraculously. However, again I heard that whisper that I was going to descend into this "valley of the shadow of death," yet I would know His presence there. God wouldn't let me go there without something redemptive in mind. Right? I also told myself that if God removed the cancer at the front end, I probably wouldn't appreciate it, because I have always been healthy—I would just get out of going through something hard. However, when confronted by the "go-for-the-healing" contingent, I felt some guilt for not having enough faith to *not* get treatment and surgery. Did Jesus have a disappointed look on His face too?

My former bosses and mentors, Andy and Jonathan, prayed for me, giving what turns out to have been the pivotal words. They said that God wasn't so concerned with me having enough faith to be healed, as entrusting myself to His goodness no matter what happens. Chemo wasn't a lack of faith, rather a means of waging war for my life. Andy prophesied that distilled through the suffering would be a joy and contentment with life. I felt great peace after those words. Indeed, going with the peace of the Lord, and not fear or guilt, became a refrain. The Lord would heal me—he would heal my wounds after surgery. My well-meaning, "faith-filled" friends calmed down after a while and got on board to stay.

Oh Lord, be the power that drives these drugs and the precision that guides the scalpel. Because here I go into that valley.

Treatment

February 21. Chemotherapy begins
There's only one printable word in a seminary paper for how chemo felt—yuuuckk! I felt like I was being squeezed through a tube head-first. I got a taste of being a human pin-cushion before treatment started with all manner of tests and scans. An old friend, from Kansas City, Ann, went with me to my

first treatment. Another friend, Renee, went to all the others. Letting friends into my lack of control and mess was a notable break from the self-sufficient, contemplative loner I'd usually been. Dietrich Bonhoeffer's words in *Life Together* came to mind:

> The Christian needs his brother man as a bearer and proclaimer of the divine word of salvation... The Christ in his own heart is weaker than the Christ in the word of his brother; his own heart is uncertain, his brother's is sure.

The reality that I was going to lose control of my body, appearance, and ability to be of use to anyone began to set in. In this, God uncovered my core believe that I am only of value through my usefulness to others. I feared being a burden and, in turn, being rejected. I tried to push people away at the beginning. I gave them an out, warning them this wasn't going to be pleasant. I was not going to be able to be present, probably a self-absorbed bore. I would understand if they wanted to reconsider the commitment they made to walk with me. To the person, they listened politely and told me to knock it off. Of course, what this really was, was the fear of being known in weakness. In reality, I loathed my weakness, believing it to be repelling. This also uncovered a disregard I had probably always had for other's vulnerability. On reflection, I see that God was working on another kind of miracle—revealing His love for me through my family of faith, right in the center of what I feared most. He was going to heal me of more than wounds from surgery.

Nobody left me. They seemed to have endless kindness, comfort, and ability to be present—God's voice, face, arms and hands. I had to sit there and take it without anything to give in return. That is hard for me. Being weak and nevertheless cared for exposed my quest up to that point, to be respected and admired, over being known and loved.

March 8. Hair loss

They said it would take 14-18 days from the first dose for the hair to fall out. It was fifteen. God was gracious to time it during a weekend. That Saturday morning, I sat in a chair over a paper sack and ran my fingers through my hair till it all had come out. It filled the sack. My roommate emerged from her bedroom to quite a sight. She declared I'd finally found the perfect hairstyle (hmm). My dear friend, Jonathan, took me out to breakfast and suggested head coverings that would look good on me. Before chemo was done, I'd lost all the hair on my body—everywhere, even in my nose. I looked into my mirror one morning and realized I looked like a turtle.

More than anything else, I had dreaded the hair loss. It pressed into my perception of being a woman. You only had to look at all the hair products in my bathroom drawer to see how much value I had given it. I felt naked for a while—more of the weakness. Again, the people around me embraced what was happening, overtime empowering me to do the same. Once the worst had happened, I relaxed and made the best of it. At least baldness and bandanas coincided with current fashion.

More thoughts during chemo

After the early days following diagnosis, I had no vertical experience of the Lord's presence—no amazing prayer times or visions. During treatment, I can count on one hand how many times I opened my Bible. The disciplines cited earlier were absent. It was through the people radiant with His presence around me, that Jesus appeared every day.

Enjoyment of reading was revived. It was God's grace I was able to focus enough. It was a rich time in terms of reading for pleasure. My amazing friend, Erin, pressed fiction books into my hand she thought I would enjoy. I ended up reading eleven books, which provided pools of enjoyment and refreshment for the imagination.

Chemo defined life as a "one day at a time" enterprise. I didn't indulge in any processing of sadness or anger about my condition. Being sad or angry wasn't going to change that I had cancer. On the other hand, there was a feeling of betrayal that something so deadly could have been growing quietly inside of me, while I moved through life comparatively without cares. I found out through reading and talking to the doctors that cancer was anarchy in the cells. It built its own vascular system, making it insensitive to stimuli. I wondered what parallels existed spiritually within me. Had I become insensitive, or hard of heart? There was a persistent worm of a belief that I had done something or didn't do so something to get cancer. I had times of fear. The movie *The Two Towers* (Lord of the Rings) animated these disturbing thoughts. There is an overpowering demonic evil army being fabricated. They were an awful sight built for intimidation and despair. When a force like that decides to set itself against you, who can stand? Their only purpose is to destroy, no softening of the heart possible—insensitivity personified. If Gandalf hadn't appeared with the dawn on the eastern horizon, the movie may have sent me into despair. My God will win. He will redeem. He will appear. Otherwise, I'm toast.

At the lowest points, vision was shrunk down to what my body felt like and was doing (or not doing). I wondered if my life was going to be anything more than a fuzzy brain, aching joints, feeling psycho with steroids, and a turtle-like appearance. There was one clear vertical experience with the Lord. Waking one morning I received what I believe was a word from Him. It wasn't a scripture, worship song, words from St. John of the Cross, Mother Teresa, Bonhoeffer, Nouwen, or a friend. I was encouraged by the words of James Bond in *Dr. No*, after he had survived a diabolical obstacle course designed by Dr. No to kill him in several different ways.

> *All he needed was an ounce of hope, an ounce of reassurance that it was still worthwhile trying to stay alive... On an instinct he felt his pulse. It was slow, but regular. The steady thump of life revived his spirits. What the hell was he worrying about? He was alive. The wounds and bruises on his body were nothing—absolutely nothing. They looked ugly, but nothing was broken. Inside the torn envelope, the machine was quietly, solidly ticking over... Get moving! Clean yourself and wake up! (Fleming, 205)*

There may be poison and a cocktail of drugs in my system. I may be hairless and have a puffy moon face. But my heart was still beating like it should. I could still walk, talk, and tell you who I was. I could tell you who you were, and where I was going. Overall, I was OK, good to go. The Lord had given some light-hearted perspective.

Scalpel Meets Skin

July 22. Surgery
This was the day I had been steadily progressing toward for six months and it was almost anticlimactic. Friends gathered the night before to lay hands on me and pray. Scans showed the chemo had been effectual. It was certain I would lose a quarter of my breast. The lymph nodes may still have to be removed. They'd only know by looking at them. I felt peaceful, even cheerful as they moved my gurney into the operating room.

They did have to remove the lymph nodes—twenty-six of them on my left side. Dr. Faddis thought he got all of the cancer. My companions, seen and unseen, were around all the time, cleaning up my messes, while effects of anesthesia moved through my system. The time following surgery moved rapidly. I mended quickly and without incident. In my spirit I was straining forward, on tip-toe. A PET scan was scheduled, an objective snapshot of what relationship my body did or did not have with cancer.

September 29. "NED"

NED means "No Evidence of Disease." This was the result of the PET scan, the most sensitive of the scans. When the nurse told me, I felt a big weight roll off. I still had to be stuck with a needle and given a dose of chemo (small this time), but for the first time I was grinning. I had become calibrated in optimism, believing I would be ultimately all right, but not surprised if there was a spot somewhere else. A clear scan left me light-headed and dazed by God's graciousness. There was great rejoicing among the faithful friends and family. I had a realization that they had too been transformed by the journey with me. Going on this pilgrimage with me was as much about their formation, as mine.

Living with uncertainty

I'm realizing that I have had a tendency to try to wrap things up, and cap questioning and doubting off with any redemptive answers I perceive. There's nothing inherently wrong with that approach, except that I can miss out on the meaning of the journey or pilgrimage by hurrying to the finish. At present, I'm feeling much more like myself, returning to a normal structure and rhythm. Yet, uncertainty continues, and will for the foreseeable future. Checking my body for cancer with scans and blood-tests is going to be a part of my life for years.

A prayer life has resumed. With all the major treatment behind me, I'm also feeling well enough to begin processing the irretrievable losses. More that has been attached to my identity, as a woman, has been altered. One of my breasts has been maimed. The chemotherapy moved me into menopause. I'm feeling the sadness from the losses both represent. I'll be getting some help to process the grief. As much as I would like to provide answers, I'll leave these matters partly unwrapped and uncapped, as I'm still walking through it.

Reflections

Transforming grace
There have been two main shifts during the last year, bringing overall widening and deepening within my spiritual life: One has been the focus on community; God relating to me through the people walking with me, and me allowing it to happen. Following that shift was a deeper reckoning with weakness, giving place to suffering in the process of transformation.

The cultivation of intimacy with Christ through the disciplines that had been so prominent in the past had been mostly individual in character. The horizontal or community dimension was given its due nod, but the focus was on the individual union with Christ, and how I changed in the process. In relationships, the role I played was of helper/servant, rarely the one receiving. However, illness overturned that dynamic. My union with Christ was through my companions. As Bonhoeffer said, "the Word of Christ" was stronger in them and they were His provision for me. In my spiritual life, the role of the body of Christ had not been as opened up as it is now. Surrendering to a season of receiving has brought more rest to my spiritual life.

Weakness and suffering had little place in my spirituality prior to being treated for cancer. When I had meditated on the humanity of Jesus, I had never thought of Him getting sick or injured. He had a job to do and, without consideration, I assumed God had kept Him from physical affliction until the passion. (And I went through all my systematic theology classes assuming that!) I had seen suffering as the result of sin, or an "educational occasion" in the words of Dr. Tiersma-Watson. Aside from the pain of the woundings of my soul that I sought healing for, times of suffering were more like a test to be passed, shed, and moved on from. However, entering into a suffering that I couldn't shed changed those assumptions and how I related to God.

Pastor John Wimber, a key contributor and overseer of the Vineyard movement (who also had cancer) said about walking through the valley of the shadow of death: "...it's frightening. Its uncertainties keep you alert to every changing scenario."

The threat of the unknown can be overwhelming. I had to embrace the truth that I could not control or plan my life. God is accomplishing His work in me, even through suffering. He is my peace.

Epilogue

God's plan for my life?

Finally, I don't believe that God planned for me to get cancer as part of a scripted drama or that my affliction had some purpose in itself; it only has meaning as it is redeemed by Christ on the Cross. Things are a complex web of circumstances with many agents playing a role. God did not miraculously intervene and deliver me from the journey, and I'll never know why. He delivers us from evil, but not from going through the "shadow of death." Still, I arrive into today trusting he is powerfully present within me and through others when I suffer and walk through that valley. He suffers with me as he did during His life, in Gethsemane and on the Cross. The power of His presence within and without will "restore my soul" and uphold me as I continue to walk in uncertainty and grief.

Appendix II

Scriptures of Healing, Hope, and Community

Recommended: Select Psalms of Lament - 3, 6, 13, 22, 25, 28, 30, 31, 32, 34, 40, 41, 42, 63, 102, 142. The book of Luke is filled with evidence of God's healing.

Isaiah 38: 16b-20
You restored me to health and let me live. Surely it was for my benefit that I suffered such anguish. In your love you kept me from the pit of destruction; you have put all my sins behind your back. For the grave cannot praise you, death cannot sing your praise; those who go down to the pit cannot hope for your faithfulness. The living, the living—they praise you, as I am doing today; parents tell their children about your faithfulness.

Psalm 103:2-5
Praise the Lord, my soul; all my inmost being, praise his holy name. Praise the Lord, my soul, and forget not all his benefits—who forgives all your sins and heals all your diseases, who redeems your life from the pit and crowns you with love and compassion, who satisfies your desires with good things so that your youth is renewed like the eagle's!

Psalm 116:1-4
I love the Lord, for he heard my voice; he heard my cry for mercy. Because he turned his ear to me, I will call on him as long as I live. The cords of death entangled me, the anguish

of the grave came over me; I was overcome by distress and sorrow. Then I called on the name of the Lord: "Lord, save me!"

Psalm 121:1-4
A song of ascents.
I lift up my eyes to the mountains—where does my help come from? My help comes from the Lord, the Maker of heaven and earth. He will not let your foot slip—he who watches over you will not slumber; indeed, he who watches over Israel will neither slumber nor sleep.

1 Peter 2:24
"He himself bore our sins" in his body on the cross, so that we might die to sins and live for righteousness; "by his wounds you have been healed."

Romans 8:11
And if the Spirit of him who raised Jesus from the dead is living in you, he who raised Christ from the dead will also give life to your mortal bodies becauseof his Spirit who lives in you.

Matthew 15:29-30
Jesus left there and went along the Sea of Galilee. Then he went up on a mountainside and sat down. Great crowds came to him, bringing the lame, the blind, the crippled, the mute and many others, and laid them at his feet; and he healed them.

James 5:14-15
Is anyone among you sick? Let them call the elders of the church to pray over them and anoint them with oil in the name of the Lord. And the prayer offered in faith will make the sick person well; the Lord will raise them up. If they have sinned, they will be forgiven.

Psalm 116:5-9
The Lord is gracious and righteous; our God is full of compassion. The Lord protects the unwary; when I was brought low, he saved me. Return to your rest, my soul, for the Lord has been good to you. For you, Lord, have delivered me from death, my eyes from tears, my feet from stumbling, that I may walk before the Lord in the land of the living.

Psalm 121:5-8
The Lord watches over you—the Lord is your shade at your right hand; the sun will not harm you by day, nor the moon by night. The Lord will keep you from all harm—he will watch over your life; the Lord will watch over your coming and going both now and forevermore.

Luke 8:42b-48
As Jesus was on his way, the crowds almost crushed him. And a woman was there who had been subject to bleeding for twelve years, but no one could heal her. She came up behind him and touched the edge of his cloak, and immediately her bleeding stopped. "Who touched me?" Jesus asked. When they all denied it, Peter said, "Master, the people are crowding and pressing against you." But Jesus said, "Someone touched me; I know that power has gone out from me."

Then the woman, seeing that she could not go unnoticed, came trembling and fell at his feet. In the presence of all the people, she told why she had touched him and how she had been instantly healed. Then he said to her, "Daughter, your faith has healed you. Go in peace."

Luke 8:41,42a, 49-50; 52-55
...a man named Jairus, a synagogue leader, came and fell at Jesus' feet, pleading with him to come to his house because his only daughter, a girl of about twelve, was dying....

While Jesus was still speaking, someone came from the house of Jairus, the synagogue leader. "Your daughter is dead," he said. "Don't bother the teacher anymore." Hearing this, Jesus said to Jairus, "Don't be afraid; just believe, and she will be healed."
… Meanwhile, all the people were wailing and mourning for her. "Stop wailing," Jesus said. "She is not dead but asleep." They laughed at him, knowing that she was dead. But he took her by the hand and said, "My child, get up!" Her spirit returned, and at once she stood up. Then Jesus told them to give her something to eat.

Ephesians 3: 14-19
For this reason I kneel before the Father, from whom every family in heaven and on earth derives its name. I pray that out of his glorious riches he may strengthen you with power through his Spirit in your inner being, so that Christ may dwell in your hearts through faith. And I pray that you, being rooted and established in love, may have power, together with all the Lord's holy people, to grasp how wide and long and high and deep is the love of Christ, and to know this love that surpasses knowledge—that you may be filled to the measure of all the fullness of God.

Psalm 42:9-11
I say to God my Rock, "Why have you forgotten me? Why must I go about mourning, oppressed by the enemy?" My bones suffer mortal agony as my foes taunt me, saying to me all day long, "Where is your God?" Why, my soul, are you downcast? Why so disturbed within me? Put your hope in God, for I will yet praise him, my Savior and my God.

Psalm 61: 2-4
From the ends of the earth I call to you, I call as my heart grows faint; lead me to the rock that is higher than I. For you

have been my refuge, a strong tower against the foe. I long to dwell in your tent forever and take refuge in the shelter of your wings.

Psalm 71: 5-7
For you are my hope; O Lord God, you are my confidence from my youth. By you I have been sustained from my birth; You are he who took me from my mother's womb; my praise is continually of you. I have become a marvel to many, for you are my strong refuge (NASB).

Jeremiah 29:11
"For I know the plans I have for you," declares the Lord, "plans to prosper you and not to harm you, plans to give you hope and a future…"

Jeremiah 30:17
…But I will restore you to health and heal your wounds,' declares the Lord, 'because you are called an outcast, Zion for whom no one cares.'

Psalm 30:2
Lord my God, I called to you for help, and you healed me.

Psalm 31:24
Be of good courage, and he shall strengthen your heart, all you that hope in the LORD (NKJV).

Psalm 86:5
You, Lord, are forgiving and good, abounding in love to all who call to you.

Psalm 107:20
He sent out his word and healed them; he rescued them from the grave.

1 Peter 1:3-5
Blessed be the God and Father of our Lord Jesus Christ, who according to His great mercy has caused us to be born again to a living hope through the resurrection of Jesus Christ from the dead, to obtain an inheritance which is imperishable and undefiled and will not fade away, reserved in heaven for you who are protected by the power of God through faith for a salvation ready to be revealed in the last time...(NASB)

Psalm 30: 3-5
O LORD, You have brought up my soul from Sheol; you have kept me alive, that I would not go down to the pit. Sing praise to the LORD, you His godly ones, and give thanks to His holy name. For His anger is but for a moment, His favor is for a lifetime; weeping may last for the night, but a shout of joy comes in the morning... (NASB)

Psalm 56:13
For you have delivered me from death and my feet from stumbling, that I may walk before God in the light of life.

Matthew 5:4
Blessed are those who mourn, for they will be comforted.

Psalm 26:3
...for I have always been mindful of your unfailing love and have lived in reliance on your faithfulness.

Colossians 2:15
And having disarmed the powers and authorities, he made a public spectacle of them, triumphing over them by the cross.

Psalm 34 (all) Excerpt: v. 4-7
I sought the Lord, and he answered me; he delivered me from all my fears. Those who look to him are radiant; their faces are

never covered with shame. This poor man called, and the Lord heard him; he saved him out of all his troubles. The angel of the Lord encamps around those who fear him, and he delivers them.

Psalm 16 (all) Excerpt: v. 9-11
Therefore my heart is glad and my tongue rejoices; my body also will rest secure, because you will not abandon me to the realm of the dead, nor will you let your faithful one see decay. You make known to me the path of life; you will fill me with joy in your presence, with eternal pleasures at your right hand...

Lamentations 3:21-23
Yet this I call to mind and therefore I have hope: Because of the Lord's great love we are not consumed, for his compassions never fail. They are new every morning; great is your faithfulness.

1 Corinthians 15:51-57 (all) Excerpt: last paragraph
It was sin that made death so frightening and law-code guilt that gave sin its leverage, its destructive power. But now in a single victorious stroke of life, all three—sin, guilt, death—are gone, the gift of our Master, Jesus Christ. Thank God (MSG).

Isaiah 53:4-5
Surely he took up our pain and bore our suffering, yet we considered him punished by God, stricken by him, and afflicted. But he was pierced for our transgressions, he was crushed for our iniquities; the punishment that brought us peace was on him, and by his wounds we are healed.

2 Corinthians 12:9
But he said to me, "My grace is sufficient for you, for my power is made perfect in weakness." Therefore I will boast

all the more gladly about my weaknesses so that Christ's power may rest on me.

Psalm 16:8
I keep my eyes always on the LORD. With him at my right hand, I will not be shaken.

Luke 9:1
When Jesus had called the Twelve together, he gave them power and authority to drive out all demons and to cure diseases...

* There have been minor adjustments in capitalization on NASB verses.

Appendix III

God's Truth Destroys Cancerous Lies

Cancerous lies	God's Truth
I am damaged goods now, marred, disfigured… No one will desire me.	*I am my beloved's, and his desire is for me…* (Song of Sol. 7:10). **Reflection:** Do not the scars of Jesus make Him more beautiful? If the King of Kings and Lord of Lords calls you desirable, there is no argument.
God wants to punish me. My sickness is God's judgment.	"*…if anyone is in Christ, the new creation has come: The old has gone, the new is here! All this is from God, who reconciled us to himself through Christ and gave us the ministry of reconciliation: that God was reconciling the world to himself in Christ, not counting people's sins against them. And he has committed to us the message of reconciliation* (2 Cor. 5:18-19). **Reflection:** God doesn't punish His children with sickness: that would be a kingdom divided against itself. He taught us to pray, "Your kingdom come, Your will be done."

Cancerous lies	God's Truth
I brought this on myself through bad eating, drinking, and behavior.	*Who then is the one who condemns? No one. Christ Jesus who died—more than that, who was raised to life—is at the right hand of God and is also interceding for us* (Rom. 8:34). *For all have sinned and fall short of the glory of God, and all are justified freely by his grace through the redemption that came by Christ Jesus (*Rom 3:23-24). **Reflection:** Behavior has consequences, but God's love is stronger and more powerful. He is mighty to save.
I must earn my healing	*For it is by grace you have been saved, through faith—and this is not from yourselves, it is the gift of God (Eph. 2:8)* **Reflection:** You didn't earn God's love, and healing is an expression of His love.
Now, I'll end up alone. No one will want to marry me. I'm too big of a risk.	*God places the lonely in families; he sets the prisoners free and gives them joy* (Ps. 68:6). **Reflection:** The right man will appreciate your journey and it won't be an issue.
My dreams cannot come true now.	*Take delight in the LORD, and he will give you the desires of your heart.* (Ps. 37:4) **Reflection:** God delights in doing what seems impossible to us. Every good and perfect gift comes from the Father of lights
The enemy is out to destroy me. He is too strong for me.	*Greater is he who is in you than he who is in the world* (1 Jn. 4:4b). **Reflection:** God invites us to draw near to Him and He will draw near to us, and if we resist the enemy, he will flee.

God's Truth Destroys Cancerous Lies

Cancerous lies	God's Truth
Because I am too weak to read or pray, I will lose this battle.	*In the same way, the Spirit helps us in our weakness. We do not know what we ought to pray for, but the Spirit himself intercedes for us through wordless groans* (Rom. 8:26). **Reflection:** God has planted you in a community. Lean on them and *especially* lean on Him.
Can God really heal something as devastating as cancer?	*And if the Spirit of him who raised Jesus from the dead is living in you, he who raised Christ from the dead will also give life to your mortal bodies because of his Spirit who lives in you.* (Rom. 8:11). **Reflection:** All things, including cancer, bow to the One who created the heavens and earth.
I don't feel God's presence. I am utterly alone. I don't know where he is.	*Neither height nor depth, nor anything else in all creation, will be able to separate us from the love of God that is in Christ Jesus our Lord* (Rom. 8:39). **Reflection:** It's not a matter of feeling, but fact: God is ever with us and in us.
No one knows what I'm going through.	*For we do not have a high priest who is unable to empathize with our weaknesses, but we have one who has been tempted in every way, just as we are—yet he did not sin* (Heb. 4:15). **Reflection:** Jesus' friends scatter. The Cross looms. Think hands. Think big nails. That's pain! He does know what we're going through even unto death.

Cancerous lies	God's Truth
Cancer is my new identity. I am named by it.	*The nations will see your vindication, and all kings your glory; you will be called by a new name that the mouth of the LORD will bestow* (Is. 62:2). **Reflection:** No illness is our identity and at all times God names us and is the informer of who we are.
As a believer, you are dishonoring God when you show your weakness. It's better to keep to yourself when you aren't doing well.	*Blessed are those who mourn for they will be comforted* (Mt. 5:4). **Reflection:** God knows we must grieve our losses. Jesus wept.

Appendix IV

Resources for Group Leaders/ Facilitators

We created this book to be used in a group setting or by individuals. We have found that in most cases healing is accelerated and supported in community. So, if possible, we encourage you to share this journey with others. There are many ways to implement this book. Below are a few suggestions.

Scheduling
- Individuals: reading, praying and journaling on a regular annual cycle
- Group: As a 1-day intensive (8-10 hours plus breaks and meals)
- Group: Divided over 2 Saturdays
- Group: Over 6 weeks (2-hour sessions)

Group Size
- Any size the facilitator is comfortable with: 2–20, or more
- A very large group could also break into smaller groups for discussion and prayer

Structure
- For weekly meetings, it's helpful to have members read through the sessions before the group meets. The Session Review discussion questions can be integrated into the sharing/teaching of the material, or saved until the end.
- The order of elements in the Session Review can be switched and you can add, delete, or reword the questions.
- Leader/Facilitator should bring as many personal anecdotes as possible to the session discussion.

Session Review Sample:

Questions for Discussion & Reflection

Usually there are questions relating to the session or thematic discussion points. If you are not in a group setting you can journal these questions and your answers.

Prayer
A different prayer for each session is supplied. Suggestions are given for leader to begin prayers by reading them out loud in short phrases with group participants repeating. In two sessions, praying in pairs is suggested.

Journal
Scriptures and reflection topics are supplied for journaling.

Further Suggestions For group Facilitation:

<u>A Critical Reminder</u>: Group members need to honor confidentiality. What is shared in the group stays in the group!

If you are facilitating *More Hope!*, the following are some suggestions for you to adapt as best fits your gathering.

- Be creative! Adapt the materials to your unique group. Feel free to bring fresh ideas to how you present the material.

- Always leave room for the Holy Spirit. Don't see discussion points as items that must be checked off a list, feel free to add or subtract.

- Keep to times agreed upon for each session. Respect the time constraints of those who attend.

- Open with worship and prayer.

- During the week pray for the participants.

- Review the materials for each week ahead of time. Answer the questions yourself.

- Have the group participants take turns reading the testimony excerpts from the women who are quoted in each session.

- Please don't tell a person that they will "live and not die." Direct them to what God says in Scripture. Encourage them with God's identity as healer. Leave it to God to speak the definitive healing word.

- Beginning in Session One, encourage group members to share their stories. Suggest that as various women's stories are read, that they consider how their own stories relate to those represented in *More Hope!*

- On the "Time to Connect to Hope," which is repeated each week, give the participants the opportunity to connect hope with that session's theme. Give participants a moment to jot down what God shows them in the "Journal" section.

- Let God be the counselor. You are a facilitator not a psychologist. If a person needs additional help, refer them to trusted Christian counselors in your area. Sometimes one needs pastoral counseling in an individual setting as well. Consider having a list of tested mentors and groups that can provide additional support.

- In the sharing time following the listening prayer exercise, make sure to affirm each sharer's ability to hear God's voice. Bless each one and the healing words they received from the Lord.

- ONE OF THE MOST IMPORTANT THINGS YOU CAN CONVEY to each member of your group whether large or small is that God has a different healing journey for each of them. The destination is the same: wholeness, abundant life, joy, peace and an unhindered relationship with God and with others. How God gets us there is tailored to our temperament and history. Encourage them not to compare themselves to another. Some people hear from God more readily and easily, some are visibly touched by His presence. Encourage them not to doubt that God is working with and in them. Consider: The healing work of God is sometimes obvious immediately, but our restoration unfolds over a lifetime. Embrace the discovery process with Him!

EMBRACING LIFE MINISTRIES

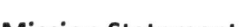

Mission Statement
Our **mission** is to help people realize the abundant life available in Christ by providing practical tools, healing seminars and equipping programs that revive hope, reclaim authority and restore true identity in Christ.

Our **vision** is to see our resources available to the Church worldwide for her healing, equipping and transformation.

For more information and other resources, contact us:

By Post
Embracing Life Ministries
1443 E. Washington Blvd. #635
Pasadena, California 91104-2650

Online
www.embracinglife.us
info@embracinglife.us

Phone
626-798-7398

Additional Resources

Embracing Life Series (ELS) – A 14-session healing discipleship series for persons with life-altering conditions of all kinds. (Also works as a discipleship resource for churches.)

Breaking Free… from the spirit of death – Exposes the source of destructive influences in one's life—the spirit of death—offering counsel and prayers for getting free and living out the abundant life Jesus promises.

More Life! Breaking Free…from the spirit of death: Guidebook Edition – Based on the *Breaking Free*…text, this booklet offers clear, practical, leader's notes, interactive questions and prayers for group participation.

More Glory! God's Healing Voice for Shame and Self-hatred – This booklet for individual or group use offers authentic hope for Christians struggling with shame, self-hatred, and hearing God's voice.

Other Resources

Damascus Road (DVD) – A TBN-produced interview with Jonathan Hunter featuring his near-death experience (NDE) and entry into faith in Jesus Christ.

Check online (www.embracinglife.us) regularly for new downloadable support resources for your groups and other materials.

www.ingramcontent.com/pod-product-compliance
Ingram Content Group UK Ltd.
Pitfield, Milton Keynes, MK11 3LW, UK
UKHW022215230426
12048UKWH00016BA/868